SOTHIS PRESS

Sothis Press aims to completely reimagine the public domain book with an emphasis on universal access to captivatingly designed print editions. We believe that technology will enable every single book ever published to be perpetually accessible in beautiful print form. Sothis is beauty in ubiquity.

www.sothis.press
1 Waterhouse Square, London, EC1N 2ST

Effects of Borax and Boracic Acid on the Human System

Oscar Liebreich

SOTHIS PRESS

ISBN 978-1-0365-1910-0

Effects of Borax and Boracic Acid on the Human System is in the public domain.

EFFECTS OF

BORAX AND BORACIC ACID

ON THE HUMAN SYSTEM.

BY

DR. OSCAR LIEBREICH,

O. Ö. PROFESSOR DER UNIVERSITÄT BERLIN, UND GEHEIMER MEDICINALRATH.

BERLIN, 1899.

(TRANSLATED FROM THE GERMAN.)

PRICE TWO SHILLINGS.

INDEX.

A

EFFECTS OF BORAX AND BORACIC ACID ON THE HUMAN SYSTEM.

Introduction.

TO judge of the salutary or harmful effect of Borax and Boric Acid on the human organism was formerly a matter of extreme difficulty, since, apart from their technical application, these substances were used for medical purposes only, never for hygienic purposes. Much as in the case of various other remedies, inexact observations and exaggerated laudation only helped to keep up the current prejudice against the preparations, and to strengthen the fear of their harmful influence. In our own time, however, the relation subsisting between the human organism and Borax and Boric Acid has become a matter of greater importance, since these substances are now used as admixtures to food. And the question whether they are really inimical to the constitution is now a supremely important one.

Borax and Boric Acid natural substances.

Borax and Boric Acid are natural mineral substances, found either as such, only requiring purification, or else variously combined with other substances. First of all must be named Boronatrocalcite, which is found in Chili, then Stassfurtite, Pinnoite, Datolite, a combination of Borate of Calcium with Silicate of Calcium, Lüneburgit, Pandermite, etc. For purposes of historical study the most interesting is *Tincal*, a raw crystallised Borax, which is found in Asia, Tartary, and Thibet, in the bed of dried-up lakes. Similar lakes have been discovered in North America, and they too now form a source from which Borax is obtained. Boric Acid is produced from Borax, or obtained from the Solfatares of Tuscany.

Historical notes.

The most ancient name for Borax is supposed to have been *Chrysocolla*, but whether this designation applied to Borax or not is by no means certain, and hence no weight can be attached to all that has been said and written about the effect of Chrysocolla on man.

The name Borax seems to be met with first in the 10th century among the Arabs. At that time Borax was used exclusively for soldering, but the Chinese are known to have employed it in the smelting process. Early in the 15th century Borax was introduced into Europe, and a century later its therapeutic application commenced; but, though carried far and wide by

Venetian traders, it remained a secret substance. Tincal brought from Persia was subjected to a refining process in Venice. Not before 1749 was its nature brought to light by REUSS. Shortly afterwards it was found in other places, and when in 1808 DAVY discovered the element Boron chemical elucidation of the Borax combinations soon followed.

Introduction of Boric preparations into medicine, and false application.

In the 18th century Boric Acid was introduced by HOMBERG as *Sal sedativum*, though possibly it may have been known to the alchemist BECHER as early as 1675. Both Boric Acid and Borax were early employed for therapeutic purposes. When, about the middle of the 16th century, Borax began to be used systematically in medicine, a quality was ascribed to it to which assuredly it cannot lay claim, viz., stimulation of labour pains. Distinguished physicians contradicted the assertion from the first, but it was not finally disproved until modern times. Other qualities were also claimed for Borax; it was said to excite menstruation, to be a remedy for cramp, for hæmorrhage, and paralysis. Even in diarrhœa and dysentery Boric Acid and Borax were given, so that both were considered to be drastic remedies. These manifold uses and the wrong views held with regard to the effects of Borax, can only be explained by the old custom of never prescribing a single remedy by itself, but always in mixture with others.

Confutation of prejudices.

We owe the first decisive confutation of all these prejudices to a prize essay written in 1845 for the Medical Faculty of the Munich University. The theme was as follows:—

> "The pharmacological qualities of Borax and of Boric Acid are to be brought out as clearly as possible by comparison and examination of all the facts at disposal, as well as by physiological and chemical experiments, with a view to showing the changes wrought by these remedies in the organic functions and mixtures."

In his prize essay LUDWIG BINSWANGER[1] proved that Boric Acid is not toxic, and he concluded:—

> "That Boric Acid in medical doses being totally indifferent to the organism should no longer be employed therapeutically, and that Borax, though analogous to, yet much weaker in its action than, bicarbonate of soda, should be subordinated to the latter, except as a solvent of uric acid, for which purpose it is more efficacious."

When once the innocuousness of Boric Acid was thus made known, it was not long before PIDOUX's and TROUSSEAU's opinion of its irritating and astringent effect was confuted. Thus it seemed that Borax was to be excluded from medicine. But before long it was recognised to possess antiseptic qualities, and further observation proved that, contrary to earlier views, Borax and Boric Acid exercise a soothing influence on the mucous membranes, even in the most sensitive places, and also on inflammatory membrane. To give an example: Boric Acid mixed with ground coffee is recommended and widely used as a remedy for cold in the head, *i.e.*, for inflamed mucous membrane of the nose. The soothing and antiseptic effect of Borax and Boric Acid caused them to be introduced into surgery. Antiseptic treatment with Boric Acid, as first tried by LISTER[2], GODLEE, and others, has been generally adopted, especially by LEONARD CANE[3], who has described numerous cases of wounds that healed normally and without irritation or inflammation after the application of a solution of Boric Acid. He sums up:—"It is an antiseptic which neither irritates nor inflames, and thus enables the natural healing process to take place without interruption." This explains that in purulent otitis too, the Boric Acid treatment introduced by BEZOLD[4] in 1887, is universally acknowledged the best. In modern internal therapeutics, Borax finds employment. It is of special interest that Borax, the mildest of alkalis, acts as a solvent of uric acid in gouty affections (as was proved by BINSWANGER), and also as a soothing agent on bladder and kidney. These therapeutical uses must be cited, since they prove the innocuousness of Borax internally applied, thus disproving many assertions to the contrary.

Recognition of new qualities.

Of course, one must not overlook the fact that idiosyncrasy may occur. What we call idiosyncrasy is when a very small minority of mankind show peculiar abnormal symptoms after the introduction of certain substances into the system. This idiosyncrasy occurs, not only after taking chemical substances, but frequently even after eating certain articles of food. It is generally known that various skin affections, accompanied by fever, may occur after strawberries or crayfish have been eaten. Many remedies, for instance quinine, iodide of potassium, etc., produce similar symptoms. Yes, even rhubarb, which is borne perfectly by many hundreds of thousands, in some solitary cases brings out great blisters on the skin. However, in the Borax and Boric Acid treatment, idiosyncrasy has never been specially noticeable. Opportunity of observing it was given in the treatment of epilepsy, treated by large doses of Borax instead of by large doses of bromide of potassium. GOWERS[5] gave 0·91 gramme daily for two years, and afterwards (it is not said how long)

Idiosyncrasy.

3·62 grammes daily, whereupon a psoriasis-eruption on the skin ensued. The same condition set in after eight months in another case of epilepsy. With the exception of these epileptic cases, no similar occurrences have been observed.

Similar observations were made in cases described by J. Jameson Evans.[6] After 1·8 grammes per day, increased to 3·6 grammes per day, dermatitis set in; in another case the nails became diseased and the hair fell out. But the author himself acknowledges that he could not be absolutely certain that no syphilitic disease was present. But these doses greatly exceed the doses employed in the preservation of food. Probably Sophia Grumpelt's case, in which she irrigated the rectum with a solution of a tea-spoonful (28 decigrammes) of Boric Acid in a pint of water, belongs to this category. For, she adds, that she has often irrigated the rectum of children with a similar solution without any untoward effect. In the external application of Boric Acid also, experience has proved that too concentrated solutions may produce eczema. Danger has been noticed more particularly where large quantities of a solution of Boric Acid were injudiciously injected into cavities of the body. In the majority of such cases that are known, only the percentage and not the quantity of the injected fluid has been stated, so that it is impossible to estimate the doses, but it is certain that they must have been large ones. To prove how useless such accounts are for scientific purposes, the following two cases of Molodenkow[8] may be quoted:—

> I. The patient was a female, aged 25, with serous exudative pleurisy. Her pleural cavity was tapped, and subsequently washed out with a 5 per cent. solution of Boric Acid. Soon after the operation vomiting ensued, which increased violently towards evening, pulse small and weak. The following day erythema set in, commencing with the face, and spreading over the back; pulse scarcely appreciable, continuous vomiting. Three days after the operation, the erythema having spread to the thighs, and the other symptoms being unchanged, the patient succumbed, consciousness being complete to the last, only visual disturbance being complained of. Unfortunately no autopsy was made.

> II. Female patient, 16 years old, with lumbar vertebral kyphosis and burrowing abscess of the right nates. Puncture of the abscess with continuous irrigation by means of a 5 per cent. Boric Acid solution. Half-an-hour later vomiting (in this case, as well as in the former one, no chloroform had been given) which continued,

then debility, pulse hardly appreciable, and after two days an erythema beginning with the face, singultus, and death. The post-mortem was almost negative, except for some extravasations on the inner surface of the pericardium; immediate cause of death, paralysis of the heart.

Similar accidents are recorded, for instance by LEMOINE,[9] Professeur à la Faculté de Médecine de Lille, who injected a 4 per cent. solution into the pleura several times in succession. Apart from the fact that the quantity of the irrigating fluid is not mentioned, the author himself confesses that necessary precautions were omitted. As in this case, so in MOLODENKOW's cases, it is obvious that the cause of death may have been other than the Boric Acid solution. Hence those authors are in error, who endeavour to prove the danger of Boric Acid by cases such as the above. Wherever the doses are stated, it can be seen that excessively large overdoses have been employed. Thus BRUZELIUS[10] describes a case in which a male patient, of 23 years of age, was given 56 to 60 grammes in 1½ litres of water twice a day as an enema, eleven days in succession. On the eleventh day serious symptoms, nausea, pain in the nose and in the pharynx, vertigo, and some skin affection set in, pulse feeble. Similar disturbances were observed in the case of a woman of 62, related by WARFWINGE,[11] after fifteen days' treatment with daily enemas of 300 grammes of 2½ per cent. solution, *i.e.*, about 15 grammes Boric Acid per day. Both patients recovered after the enemas had been discontinued. Both these cases might more appropriately be cited as a proof that even overdoses do no lasting harm. Similar cases, described by HOGNER,[12] RASCH,[13] and WELCH,[14] are on record; it is true they are not quite so lucid in character, the pathological condition of the patients rendering a decisive opinion difficult.

It is not the medicinal use of Borax and Boric Acid that has given so great a prominence to the question as to whether these substances are injurious to the organism, but rather their application to the purposes of food preservation.

Boric Acid causes no change in the blood.

At ordinary temperature Boric Acid belongs to the weakest acids known. Even taste can hardly detect its acidity. How extremely slight its action is on organic tissues is seen by the blood. Two per cent solutions of Boric Acid do not prevent coagulation of blood; even concentrated Boric Acid, mixed freely with fresh blood, only delays and cannot prevent coagulation. In fact, Boric Acid has scarcely the character of an acid, and thus, after numerous experiments, Brücke's[15] words are fully justified:—

> If we look back on all that has been said, it is clear that, in its action on albuminous bodies, Boric Acid has no analogy with any other acid hitherto examined for this purpose, with the sole exception of carbonic acid gas. Here however, the similarity is so complete, that carbonic acid gas, apart from the qualities inherent in its gaseous condition, acts exactly like diluted Boric Acid.

Boric preparations act as preservatives on fresh material only.

Borax, on the other hand, by its reactions, proves itself to belong to the weaker alkaline combinations. Hence food, brought in contact with it, is not changed at all in its chemical constitution. If we ask how far the disinfecting power of Borax and Boric Acid goes, the answer is: that they are only very weak antiseptics. In a 4 per cent. solution of Boric Acid staphylococci retain their vitality for ten days. Even concentrated solutions can do no more than arrest growth in the case of most microbes, and hence many authors deny that Borax preparations possess any antiseptic effect. But, since this effect exists, as has been amply proved by experience, the only explanation of it is that the arrest of growth suffices to protect food from infection and decomposition. It follows from this that Boric Acid has not the power of restoring spoiled food to its former normal condition. Once decomposition has set in, Boric Acid loses its efficacy, and all it can do is to preserve fresh goods in their natural state. This is the essential distinction between boracic preparations and salicylic preparations; a valuable distinction, as it is impossible by the boracic method to restore food even when only slightly tainted. These facts, moreover, are in harmony with surgical experience; a decayed tooth for instance, which can be disinfected by every other kind of disinfectant, is not influenced by Borax. Meat and other solid substances need only be covered by boracic preparations to keep fresh. Fish treated in the same way remain wholesome, a fact proved by Liebreich[16] in 1887. Experiments with concentrated Boric Acid show that it is possible to destroy the protoplasm of the cells, but this destruction must be ascribed to the alkaline concentration and not to the specific action of Borax. Fermentation is arrested by concentrated solutions. However, these strong concentrations are not required in practice, and in fact are never employed.

Boric preparations in use for a long period of time.

The most important question in the use of preservatives for food is naturally, How do they agree with the human organism? Opposition to the use of boracic preparations has been raised, supported by the prejudices handed down from bygone times, and special stress, as already stated, has been laid upon the accidents which have happened in surgical application, and to a considerable extent upon imperfect experimental researches. From a practical point of view, this question might indeed have been considered as already decided in a favourable sense, since—*notwithstanding the fact that Borax and Boric Acid have been in use as food preservatives for a series of decades, not a single case of injury to health has been observed*, just as in the pickling and smoking of meat, to which processes no objection has ever been made, although unnecessarily large quantities of saltpetre and the empyreumatic substances such as carbolic acid and creosote, which are all used, can—unlike Borax and Boric Acid—have a toxic effect.

Since opinion as to the applicability of boracic preparations to food is divided, it will be advisable to weigh the chief points for and against, elucidating obscure points by well-planned experiments in order to be able to give a decision whether valid reasons exist for discarding the practical experience of many years, and above all, in order to make sure of the limits within which there need be no fear of injury to health.

Boric preparations non-poisonous (*See* also p. 13).

And here it may be said at once, that *boric preparations do not belong to the poisonous substances*. From nature herself we may learn that a substance which occurs constantly in many cells, as Boric Acid does, cannot be called a strong poison. It has been alleged that Boric Acid is a poison for plants, but this is the case only if the soil be over-saturated with Borax and Boric Acid. Where there is over-saturation, the effect of Borax is similar to that of many other non-poisonous mineral substances: growth is retarded or arrested. But Boric Acid is not only non-poisonous, it is a *normal constituent part of many plants*. There was a considerable stir in 1888 when BAUMERT[17] demonstrated the presence of Boric Acid in Californian wines. The first assumption was that there must be adulteration, but this proved ungrounded, for in SCHMITT'S laboratory at Wiesbaden, RIPPER had previously found Boric Acid in 1,000 different German and Foreign wines, which could not be traced to adulteration. Further, proof was brought that Boric Acid occurs in the vines themselves, and that it thus enters the wine in a natural way. It was even possible to isolate Borium as Bor-Fluor-Potassium from two litres of a pure Rissling wine. Later on BAUMERT succeeded in demonstrating the presence of Boric Acid in the leaves and the wood of various species of vine in the Freiburg district, thus incontestably proving that Boric Acid is an invariable natural ingredient of wine. Boric Acid has also been traced in the so-called wild vine or virginia creeper (*Ampelopsis quinquefolia*).

Boric Acid a normal constituent of plants.

It is true that Boric Acid does not occur as a normal ingredient of all vegetable products. There is none in cider, for instance, as Boric Acid does not occur in apples. But Boric Acid is found in water melons, and here it is probably invariable, as it was present in each of the specimens examined. Moreover, H. JAY[18] has proved that a number of plants absorb Boric Acid occasionally; he found $2\frac{1}{10}$ to $4\frac{6}{10}$ per thousand in the ash of these plants.

Now it is true that substances which have a poisonous effect on the organism in general, such as arsenous acid for instance, can now and then be absorbed by plants, but such a substance has never been demonstrated as invariably present in any one kind of plant, whilst this has been proved in the case of Boric Acid. Though this presence is interesting, since it shows that minimum quantities of Boric Acid can be taken continuously—or, as in the case of mineral waters, temporarily—without ill-effects, it must be remembered that in the preserved food question we have to deal with larger quantities, and, above all, with more continuous general use.

No cases of acute poisoning by the *internal application* of Boric Acid or Borax are known. But here it must be expressly stated once more, that resorption by the surface of wounds in the rectum or the vagina in pathological cases do not come under consideration, as the conditions of gastric and intestinal resorption are totally different. A case in point is saltpetre, which salt is not poisonous when introduced into the stomach and the intestines, but which, when introduced into a blood vessel, even in small doses, causes the phenomena of poisoning. It would not have been necessary to dwell especially on this point, were it not that this difference is not well brought out in many text-books of toxicology, and even passed over in some.

Almost all easily obtainable poisonous substances are occasionally used in attempts at suicide, and thus give opportunities to study their toxic action. Not so in the case of Borax and Boric Acid. Not a single case is to be found in medical literature. Boric Acid is often prescribed as a mouth wash or gargle, and if it were poisonous we should thus have been able to study its effects, much as, unfortunately, we have studied the effects of chlorate of potash. But, though its use is very general, no disadvantageous observation is on record. On the other hand, LEGENDRE,[19] in his "Traité pratique d'Antisepsie appliqué à la Thérapeutique et à l'Hygiène," relates that POLLI describes a case, in which a soldier swallowed 25 grammes (!) of Boric Acid by mistake, without bad results. A series of experiments were made on himself by BINSWANGER to test the effect of Boric Acid. He took 5 grains of Boric Acid fasting, noticed no effect during the forenoon, took four more doses of 5 grains each two hours apart during the afternoon, and finally the last dose at eight o'clock p.m., *i e.*, more than 18 decigrammes in all, without any other effect—as the author himself says—than that he enjoyed his supper famously. It was not until he had increased the dose tenfold that it began to disagree with him A drachm (3,654 milligrammes) was taken, without producing abnormal symptoms. It was only when a second drachm was taken, after two hours' interval, that vomiting set in. A third dose having been taken in the course of the afternoon, he again vomited; after a couple of hours however, he completely regained his normal condition.

Innocuousness even in prolonged use.

Even large doses of Boric Acid taken continuously for some length of time have not proved injurious to health. This conclusion is justified from the observations made in internal application, and some experiments on human cases. Polli[20] relates: eight persons were able to take each 2 grammes of Boric Acid dissolved in milk daily for 45 days, and 4 grammes daily for 23 days, without showing the slightest abnormal symptom. The urine passed during the period remained acid and without any sign of decomposition for a considerable time.

Binswanger's experiments on himself.

Borax, which shows an alkaline reaction, cannot be borne in such overdoses by the stomach, because alkalis have such a marked tendency to produce nausea. These experiments too, have been made on himself by Binswanger. Overdoses brought on vomiting, but no general symptoms of poisoning, although the entire Borax swallowed could not have been brought up. The author took a drachm (3,654 milligrammes) between 5 and 6 a.m. in divided doses. Up to the third dose no effect whatever was noticed, neither a rise in the skin's temperature, nor any influence on the frequency of the pulse. It was not until the fourth dose that slight tendency to nausea set in, which disappeared after an hour. When a drachm of Borax was divided into two doses and taken in the course of the morning, no inconvenience was felt for the entire day.

Doses in medicinal use.

Boric Acid has been taken therapeutically for weeks and months, in doses up to 15 decigrammes, without producing any untoward symptoms. And Borax, even in large doses, and taken during a prolonged period, has been borne without inconvenience. This is authoritatively borne out by some self-observations of Virchow,[21] who for three months kept to an alkaline diet with large doses of Borax, and found that, far from doing him harm, the treatment had a curative effect. If overdoses of Borax—*not* Boric Acid—were to be given for an undue length of time, the result, as in the case of other alkalis, would necessarily be a scorbutic condition. There has however, been no opportunity to observe such an effect.

All these large doses of Borax and Boric Acid are out of the question for hygienic purposes, but they serve to show that smaller doses can be easily borne by the organism. Nevertheless, it seemed advisable to turn to *animal experiments* for further investigation of the effects of Boric Acid, in order to have a firmer basis for forming an opinion on boracic preparations.

It is true that we cannot always draw direct inferences from animal experiments as to the effect of a substance. But the question of toxic or favourable influence may be answered with the fullest certainty from dog experiments, whilst rabbit and guinea-pig experiments lead to positive results in the feeding question.

Experiments on dogs with Boric Acid.

Dogs can bear large doses of Boric Acid. We may assume, according to NEUMANN,[22] that, with a body weight of 15 kilogrammes, 5 to 6 grammes of Boric Acid constitute the maximum dose, while larger doses may lead to diarrhœa and vomiting. For this reason dogs were fed with comparatively large doses. The animals selected were a dog weighing 12 kilo 700 grammes, and another weighing 8 kilo 530 grammes. The corresponding maximum doses would accordingly be 4·20 to 5·08 grammes for dog A, and 2·83 and 3·40 grammes for dog B. Dog A was given 3 grammes and dog B 2 grammes (*see* Appendix 1), doses varying but little from those which, applied internally, produce disturbances. On the twelfth day, in the case of dog A, and on the fifteenth in the case of dog B, vomiting set in. Though dogs are occasionally subject to vomiting after being fed with a monotonous diet, yet in this case the effect is to be considered as proceeding from the Boric Acid. After 36 days of feeding, no unfavourable change in general health had taken place. The dogs looked healthy, and, what is most important, dog A had even gained 260 grammes in weight, while the weight of dog B had undergone no appreciable change. In order to gain a basis for comparison, parallel experiments were made with bicarbonate of soda and saltpetre, both of which salts are generally considered of a more harmless nature. The doses given were the same, but the dogs were considerably heavier ones, their body weight surpassing that of the first dogs by 4 per cent. Dog D (weight 17 kilo 200 grammes) was given 3 grammes bicarbonate of soda daily for 36 days; dog E (weight 27 kilo 800 grammes) the same daily dose of saltpetre (*see* Appendix 2).

Parallel experiments with saltpetre and bicarbonate of soda.

Comparison showed that both these salts act much more powerfully on the intestinal function than Boric Acid, for both dogs passed thin liquid stools during four and five days respectively. Bicarbonate of soda had no influence on the body weight, but the *saltpetre-fed* dog showed a *loss of weight* amounting to 5 kilo 400 grammes, *i.e.*, equal to 19.4 per cent.

If the feeding-doses of Boric Acid be kept below the maximum dose, cases recorded in physiological literature prove that no disturbance whatever ensues, and my own experiments demonstrated that when a dog C was fed for 24 consecutive days with about one-third the maximum dose of Boric Acid, no untoward effects were observed (see Appendix 1), whilst at the close of the feeding period the dog had gained 370 grammes in weight. Experiments upon rabbits gave similar results. Three rabbits of 1370 grammes, 1270 grammes, and 1170 grammes weight respectively, were each given 30 centigrammes Boric Acid in 60 cubic centimetres water mixed with their food for 31 days. The animals fed willingly on the oat mash (see Appendix 3[1]), their health was undisturbed, and at the close of the feeding period they had gained in weight 30 grammes, 100 grammes, and 80 grammes respectively. Like experiments were made on three rabbits, which were given 1 decigramme Boric Acid in 60 cubic centimetres water mixed with their oat food (see Appendix 3[2]), and the result was here also an increase in weight and no disturbance in the general condition. If the gain in both feeding processes be calculated, the difference is found to be within the limit of error in this kind of investigation, and therefore admits of no inference.

As regards feeding with *Borax*, nothing certain was known on the subject of maximum doses for dogs. Occasionally 10 grammes Borax had been given in food without injury to dogs weighing 10 kilogrammes whilst in other cases small doses had been observed to produce vomiting. Experience of alkaline feeding seems to point out that Borax, as an alkali, is less well borne when introduced into the stomach, and that should it reach the intestine in its concentrated condition, symptoms of irritation must necessarily supervene. In order to decide this question, the attempt was made to give to a dog a large dose of Borax in food. GRUBER[23] had already attempted to give dogs 15 to 20 grammes, for which doses the animals showed aversion; but no general conclusions can be drawn from these experiments as to the dogs' dislike of this substance, since aversion to so large a quantity of any salt is only natural. Such large doses therefore were not made use of.

A dog of 12 kilo 200 grammes weight was given meat food with 5 grammes Borax dry per day (see Appendix 3[3]). On the sixteenth day, the dog having meanwhile gained 1 kilogramme, symptoms of violent intestinal inflammation set in and continued for five days. There was severe hæmorrhage, appetite diminished, and howling and whining indicated a condition of pain. The dosing was continued during this period. On the fifth day of illness the dog recovered and seemed quite lively. For 70 days longer it was fed with 5 grammes Borax daily, making a total of 450 grammes Borax *within 90 days*.

At the end of this period it had gained 3 kilo 400 grammes in weight! This experiment shows conclusively that Borax in too great concentration or given in substance, as was here the case, is able to call forth intestinal symptoms, but that, in spite of the phenomena of intestinal irritation, no toxic influence on the entire organism could be observed, a fact supported primarily by the increase of weight from 12 kilo 200 grammes to 15 kilo 620 grammes, *i.e.*, 2·8 per cent. *Other alkalis are not known to be so mild in their influence on the animal organism.*

Experiments on rabbits prove that even larger doses of Borax repeatedly given are well borne if the solid salt be not used. A rabbit of 2400 grammes received twice, on the first day and the fifth, the enormous dose of 5 grs. Borax mixed with 20 cubic centimetres water. The œsophageal probang was used (see Appendix 3[4]). There was not the slightest trace of any intestinal symptom.

Guinea-pigs were fed with large doses (5 decigrammes) of Borax (see Appendix 4). They were given this dose in 60 cubic centimetres water in their food every day for 95 days. The animals remained in their normal condition throughout the whole period, and at its close they had increased in weight from 425 to 436 grammes, *i.e.*, 11 grammes; from 340 to 377 grammes, *i.e.*, 37 grammes; and from 330 to 383 grammes *i.e.*, 53 grammes or 8 per cent., $9\frac{7}{10}$ per cent., and 16 per cent., respectively.

The primary result of all these experiments is, that no determined aversion of animals against Borax and Boric Acid exists. This is so far favourable, as opposition to feeding on unfamiliar substances is not infrequently met with from the start. Moreover, the experiments demonstrate the important fact of increase in weight. This last phenomenon can be found too in other feeding experiments that are recorded in medical literature, for instance in Cyon's[24] cases. A dog of 19 kilo 200 grammes gained 2 kilo 950 grammes in 19 days, a second dog of 23 kilo 700 grammes gained 1 kilo 900 grammes, and a third of 12 kilo 600 grammes gained 3 kilo 100 grammes in the same period. These figures suffice to justify the assumption that the increase in weight cannot be due to chance factors. Cage feeding is more favourable to the gain of weight than feeding in the open, and therefore it would be a mistake to imagine that feeding with boracic preparations exercises a special influence on such increase. *But certainly the conclusion is justified, that nutrition was not impaired by the admixture of the said preparations*, even if it be conceded that Cyon's dogs were in an unhealthy condition previous to his experiments. The facts brought out by these feeding experiments are important, because poisonous qualities have been attributed to Borax and Boric Acid, *whilst here we have the proof to the contrary.*

Experiments on metabolism and the assimilation of food have been undertaken with a view to forming authoritative conclusions as regards the problem of nutrition. Borax and Boric Acid were both given simultaneously in food, but the inferences drawn from the experiments cannot be subscribed to unreservedly. The investigations of GRUBER may be mentioned. He finds increased excretion of urea, and draws the following conclusion :— Metabolism.

> This experiment shows, therefore, that Borax does not "save albumen," but, that, like common salt, Glauber's salt, and other neutral salts, it causes increased excretion of water, and thus increased disintegration of albumen.

It is hardly necessary to combat this opinion, since such large quantities as were used by GRUBER do not enter into the food question. On the other hand, GRUBER's judgment is favourable to the use of Borax, inasmuch as he says :

> On the assimilation of food, Borax did not act unfavourably, for the amount of the fæces, their solid contents, and the daily amount of nitrogen contained in them, were within the average in meat feeding. No injurious effect could be observed, even in the case of the largest dose (20 grammes) given in food. Appetite too was not found diminished on the day following the experiment.

These experiments, of course, have done nothing to elucidate the problem of metabolism where Borax and Boric Acid are taken ; they only serve as an example that even overdoses of Borax are without danger.

Elaborate experiments on metabolism have been made by FORSTER.[25] An exaggerated interpretation, in the sense of condemning the use of boracic preparations, has repeatedly been given to them, whereas the author himself writes :—

> On the motion of this sub-commission, and in accordance with the drift of my report, the general commission declined to apply to the State authorities for legislative measures on the subject. (Amsterdam, 1881.)

Before experiments on metabolism can be applied to practice, criticism must be brought to bear on the inferences drawn from them, in order to decide how far they are justifiable.

In these experiments animals are brought to an equilibrium of nitrogen, *i.e.*, they are fed in such a way as to make the nitrogen introduced in food equal to the nitrogen excreted through the urine and fæces, besides the loss of nitrogen which takes place by the hair and epidermis. If unfamiliar substances are mixed with the food, and if subsequently there is an increase of nitrogen in the fæces, this has by some been assumed to mean imperfect assimilation of food. This axiom in its baldness is incorrect. FORSTER himself, who is so often wrongly cited in a sense unfavourable to the influence of Borax, has specially dwelt on the incomplete results which such experiments give, and HOPPE-SEYLER had previously expressed the same view. This cannot be expressed better than in FORSTER's own words:

> The case is by no means a simple one, and I quite understand that in the above experiments too, all the necessary investigations of details have not been made, but only the first steps taken—so to speak—on the road that has been laid out. HOPPE-SEYLER's remarks also show that the quantitative examinations and determinations of the evacuations of the bowels, as they have been carried out hitherto, are only of relative value, since they do not take into consideration the exact composition of the evacuations, but for the most part only the dry substance, nitrogen and ash, of which they are composed. In the more popular as well as in scientific works on human nutrition, we frequently meet of late with views from which it would seem as though the problem of the so-called utilisation of different food-stuffs in the human intestine had been almost completely solved since HOFFMANN's, VOIT's, and RUBNER's experiments. In another place I have registered a warning against such an assumption, and have expressed my opinion that real enlightenment on this subject may be hoped for from further experiments, for which our present investigations will form but the starting-point. This opinion is fully borne out by certain results obtained in the experiments in question.

For instance, the fæces of our series of experiments of October—November, 1882, contain in their desiccated substance the following amount of nitrogen in grammes:—

Experiment.	In "insoluble" residue.	In alcohol, etc., extract.	Total.
1	1·31	4·56	5·87
2	2·39	3·49	5·88
3	2·07	3·69	5·76

There can be no reasonable doubt that the nitrogen contained in the alcoholic etc., extracts, forms a part of combinations, originating in the juices discharged into the intestine from the interior of the body. Now if—in the above experiments—the amount of absorption of the nitrogenous substances were to be calculated from the total nitrogenous contents of the fæces, we should arrive at erroneous conclusions. Though the figures concerned are small, the error may nevertheless be quite large, for in the experiments mentioned we calculate percental amount of assimilation of the nitrogenous contents of food as follows :—

Experiment.	From the total amount of nitrogen in the fæces.	From the nitrogenous contents of the fæces treated by extraction.
1	6·7	1·5
2	8·0	3·2
3	7·5	2·7

According to the first column, the supposed amount assimilated would be three times less than in reality; on the average 7·4 against 2·5 per cent. And it is clear that the less nitrogen contained in the food taken, the greater the error.

Now Forster found the nitrogenous contents of the fæces to be considerable when Boric Acid is taken. But as only one experiment upon man was made, it was necessary to have recourse to animal experiments, which are equally conclusive in this case.

Chittenden[26] carried out three experiments on dogs in five feeding periods, the result in every case being an increase of nitrogen in the fæcal masses. My own investigations confirmed this result (*see* Appendix No. 5). It seems certain therefore, that an increase—though hardly an important one —of the nitrogenous contents of fæces, takes place when Borax or Boric Acid is taken in food.

The superficial inference, that such an increase is prejudicial to nutrition, cannot be acquiesced in, and Forster rightly judges as follows :—

On the basis of these experimental results we are justified in assuming, that the admixture of Boric Acid to food exercises a favourable influence in so far that through its being eaten with food the phenomena of putrefaction in the intestine, which ensue where a mixed diet is taken, and which, by the formation of aromatic substances in the intestine may lead to excretion of sulphuric-acid-ethers in the urine, are diminished. In fact, the above figures lead to the conclusion, that this diminution continues for some time after the supply of Boric Acid has been interrupted.

Closer observation confirms this last inference, for the diminished excretion of coupled sulphuric acids through the urine is not caused simply by the action of Borax and Boric Acid in the food during the process of digestion, but by the excretion of these substances after absorption by the stomach and intestines, Borax and Boric Acid exercising a sort of double influence on the organism. Thus, nitrogenous substances are not transformed into absorbable products of putrefaction in the intestine.

Effect on digestion and saliva. Comparison with soda and saltpetre.

Though the feeding experiments have not brought out any specially unfavourable influence on digestion where the maximum doses were not exceeded, it seemed desirable nevertheless, to examine Borax and Boric Acid in their relation to the process of *digestion*, in order to find out whether possibly they might do harm. Here too the values obtained could only be rightly judged when compared with the digestion results in presence of other salts. First of all, the saliva was subjected to examination. CHITTENDEN[27] proved that the sugar-forming power of the saliva is but slightly diminished by Boric Acid. Borax he found to have a very considerable influence; 5 per cent. brought about a diminution of 57·8 per cent. sugar.

The results given in Appendix 6 likewise demonstrate that Borax lowers the sugar-forming power. Still it may be questioned whether this diminution should not be ascribed to alkalinity. Both Table A and Table B show that carbonate of soda has a far more powerful influence, an admixture of 5 decigrammes completely suspending the saccharifying power of the saliva. Saltpetre, on the other hand, exercises no disturbing influence on the fermentative action. And as regards gastric digestion, proof could be brought that where the Borax digestion was properly directed, $\frac{1}{10}$ per cent. and $\frac{1}{4}$ per cent. did not produce any trace of disturbance (see Appendix 7[1]); $\frac{1}{2}$ per cent. caused a slight disturbance, such as always accompanies similar digestion experiments whenever the amount of common salt is largely increased by the addition of hydrochloric acid in presence of soda salts. If we bring this experiment to bear on the process of digestion in man and in animals, we find that Borax has a neutralising action, without injuring digestion, in the same way as carbonate or bicarbonate of soda. Moreover, since in gastric digestion the

Gastric digestion.

contents of the stomach are constantly being evacuated, while at the same time there is a continuous renewal of hydrochloric acid from the coats of the stomach, the experiment made outside the organism does not authorise the inference that Borax disturbs digestion. In the internal application of Borax, just as in the experiment outside the organism, the only effect to be considered is that of Boric Acid, and the difference between it and the effect of Borax must be sought in the fact that Borax, as an alkali, has a neutralising action. And that Boric Acid is by no means a poison for the digestion can be demonstrated by making the digestion experiment with internal application of Boric Acid. For this purpose quantities of from $\frac{1}{10}$ to 5 per cent. were made use of (see Appendix 7[2]). After 24 hours no undigested remains could be detected in any of the cases. The high dose of 5 per cent. Boric Acid could be used in this case, as it was soluble in the liquid at 100·4° Fahr.

Much more unfavourable were the results of the experiments with saltpetre. When $\frac{1}{10}$ per cent. was used, only about three-quarters of the albumen was digested; when the dose reached $\frac{1}{5}$ per cent., digestion began to cease (see Appendix 7[3]).

The *Pancreatic effect* too can be estimated approximately from experiments outside the organism. For this purpose a decoction of starch and solutions of Borax, Boric Acid, carbonate of soda, and nitrate of potassium were mixed with an extract of the pancreatic gland of a pig. From the figures in Appendix 8 it will be seen that *neither Borax nor Boric Acid exercises any disturbing influence on the transformation of starch into sugar.* In this respect they resemble saltpetre, whilst, on the other hand, even $\frac{1}{2}$ per cent. of carbonate of soda has a decidedly deleterious action. The power to dissolve albumen possessed by both pepsine and pancreas has been tested by KEPPLER[28] but a very short time ago, the author having previously impregnated the albumen with Borax and Boric Acid. With this experimental arrangement too, he came to the result *that the presence of Borax or Boric Acid in food does not in any way injure the chemical efficacy of the digestive ferments.* Pancreas.

In the case of other soluble ferments too, we find that Boric Acid exercises no influence whatever, and Borax has an arresting influence solely by reason of its alkaline effect. Experiments were instituted for the purpose of testing the influence of Borax, Boric Acid, carbonate of soda, and saltpetre on emulsine (see Appendix 9). We know that emulsine effects a transformation of amygdaline into oil of bitter almonds, prussic acid, and sugar. The prussic acid formed can easily be determined quantitatively. Emulsine.

In these experiments a control experiment resulted in the determination of 98⅕ per cent. With an admixture of ½ per cent. of Boric Acid, 98 per cent. were found, and with doses increasing to 5 grammes, 97½ per cent. These figures show (since such fluctuations within the limit of error may occur) that Boric Acid leaves the transformation intact. Borax, on the other hand, brings down the formation of prussic acid; 1 gramme lowers it to 16⅗ per cent., 3 grammes even to 8⅘ per cent. But it has no toxic influence on the ferment, for carbonate of soda, as an alkali, shows a much more powerful effect. This latter substance, at 1 per cent., brings down the quantity of prussic acid found to 2½ per cent. Saltpetre has certainly a more deleterious influence, and in its case the alkaline effect cannot be made responsible, as it is a neutral salt. At ½ per cent. there is a descent to 83⅘ per cent. of the calculated quantity.

It is well known that, besides this chemical action, an important factor in the digestive process is the *gastric and intestinal epithelia.* Hence any substance likely to injure the epithelium by chemical action could not but be considered injurious to the system.

Curiously enough, FORSTER's supposition that 3 per cent. Boric Acid causes disintegration of epithelium, has passed into literature, and often been repeated without any indication of its source, so that gradually the disintegration of epithelia and increased separation of intestinal mucus have come to be regarded as an established fact.

Now FORSTER (who, by the way, drew his inference from the observation of a single case) expresses himself most cautiously; his words being that these phenomena "probably" occur, and that, "for obvious reasons they cannot be completely ascertained." However, since these mere suppositions have by degrees been transformed into decided assertions, it seemed advisable to test them by means of animal experiments.

The *acid effect* of Boric Acid and the *alkaline effect* of Borax on the ciliated epithelium were then examined. The mucous membrane of the frog offers a convenient example of ciliary motion. It must be admitted that possibly its mechanical power of resistance is inferior to that of the human or mammalian ciliated epithelium; however, in our case the chief object is not to draw inferences and apply them to the human system, but rather to show that other substances, occasionally introduced into the human system, exercise a far more powerful influence on the epithelium than Borax and Boric Acid.

By using the well-known microscopic arrangement, it was possible to prove that ciliary motion is not arrested by a solution of Boric Acid, weaker than 2 to 3 per cent., whilst in the case of Borax *a 4 per cent. solution caused no diminution whatever, even after 20 minutes.* On the application of a 5 per cent. solution the motion was arrested immediately on contact with the liquid.

Naturally the questions arise: Are the values thus obtained high ones or low ones? Are they applicable to other substances also? And, Is the effect a specific one, or simply an alkaline, acid, and salt effect?

Now, it can be shown that 5 per cent. solutions of saltpetre or common salt likewise arrest the ciliary motion; therefore, the limit of the arresting power of Borax must be ascribed to the endosmotic effect of the salt, just as in the case of saltpetre or common salt. Below these limits of physical action the ciliary motion remains just as lively under the influence of Borax as of the other salts. For Boric Acid the case is similar. Here the acid re-action alone is effective. Comparatively strong solutions of Boric Acid are required to arrest ciliary motion, whereas far smaller quantities of other acids suffice for the purpose. For instance, $\frac{1}{10}$ per mille hydrochloric acid and $\frac{1}{20}$ per mille phosphoric acid are able to destroy the motion of ciliated epithelium. These investigations give clear proof that *Borax and Boric Acid cannot be considered injurious to the ciliary epithelium.*

More important than the action on the ciliated epithelium is the influence on the epithelium of the *gastro-intestinal canal.* This question can be decided by vivisection experiments. It is quite possible to examine the direct influence of Borax and Boric Acid on the living epithelium. **Action on gastro-intestinal epithelium. ciliated epithelium, Comparison with soda and saltpetre.**

Dogs were experimented on. Under narcosis, by means of morphia and ether, the stomach and intestine were laid open and irrigated for five minutes with ½, 1, 2, 3, and 5 per cent. solutions of Borax and Boric Acid respectively. For purposes of comparison, parallel experiments with solutions of common salt, saltpetre, and soda were instituted. The mucous membrane of the stomach and intestine was examined while fresh, then observed under the microscope, and re-examined later on in permanent microscopic preparations.

The results obtained will be found in the Appendices 10 to 15. the more instructive microscopic preparations being illustrated on Plates 1 and 2, Figs. 1 to 12.

The final result of this investigation is that Boric Acid, even in a 5 per cent. solution, causes no change either in the stomach or intestine. *Boric Acid exercises no injurious action whatever on the gastro-intestinal epithelium.*

Borax has a more powerful action. Up to ½ per cent. solution indeed, the gastric condition remains normal, a 1 per cent. solution causes very slight changes, the free surface of the cells is affected, *i.e.*, they become translucent, as may be observed in microscopic preparations when an alkali is added; the mucuos secretion is slightly increased, and there is an extremely small disintegration of epithelia. These cell phenomena, however, are of no biological importance, as they could only be detected after the minutest examination. Not until the solution reaches a *2 per cent. strength and upwards* does a distinct increase of mucuos secretion take place, together with the first disintegration of epithelial cells, *i.e.* a deleterious effect. The intestinal effect is milder; here too the cells become translucent, *but only distinctly so when a 3 per cent. solution is reached.* There is no disintegration of epithelia under a 5 per cent. solution.

In order to judge the effect of Borax fairly, other chemical substances occasionally introduced into the system should be drawn into the experiment. If we compare the observations in Appendix 12, we find, what is not surprising, that the prominent effect of borax is that of an alkali. This is clearly shown by the soda experiments. Even so weak a solution as 1 per cent. of soda has an injurious effect on the gastric mucous membrane, for we observe that not only are the cells rendered translucent, as in the case of Borax, but cells begin to be disintegrated. At 3 per cent. solution dilatation of the blood capillaries under the mucous membrane sets in, a phenomenon which is not observed in the application of Borax.

On the intestine the action of soda is considerably more powerful than that of Borax. At 1 per cent. solution the deleterious action commences; cells in large quantity being disintegrated, whereas a 1 per cent. Borax solution leaves the intestine intact. *In the case of saltpetre, the injurious effect on the stomach—and on the intestinal membrane too—begins at the ½ per cent. solution.* It is worthy of note, that even common salt in a 5 per cent. solution, exercises an inflammatory action on the gastro-intestinal mucous membrane. Here too, we have the proof that no other effect than an alkaline one can be ascribed to Borax, and that it has no specific injurious action of its own.

For the practical purposes of alimentation such strong solutions of Borax and Boric Acid do not come in question; but even if such should be taken, the intestinal contents would be so much diluted by the gastro-intestinal juice, by the flow of gastric juice, bile, and intestinal secretion, that the concentration would fall far below the limit value.

Small continuous doses.

BROUARDEL[29] has very justly pointed out that even small doses of chemical substances, if taken in food continuously for a long period of time, may affect health. He particularly draws attention to salicylic acid as being injurious in cases of weak or diseased kidney by its accumulation in the system. This is not so with Borax and Boric Acid. Weak and diseased kidneys bear Borax and Boric Acid particularly well; in fact, they form remedies of great value in kidney diseases, as VIRCHOW's own case shows. Moreover, in the animal experiments, there was no trace of any disturbance in the function of the kidney, so that BROUARDEL's dictum on salicylic acid cannot hold good for Borax and Boric Acid.

Borax is easily excreted from the system.

Animal experiments demonstrate further that Borax is *easily excreted* from the system, and that *no accumulation takes place.* This is clearly shown by the following experiments: Two dogs, one weighing 8 kilo 640 grammes, and the other 8 kilo, were fed for five consecutive days; dog No. 1 with Borax, and dog No. 2 with Boric Acid, the dose being 150 centigrammes daily, dissolved in 60 cubic cent. water and mixed with the ordinary food. Thirty hours were allowed to elapse after the last dose, the animals then killed, and their brain, spinal cord, blood, liver, and bone marrow chemically examined for Boric Acid without the slightest trace being found. And in rabbits, which had been fed for five consecutive days with daily doses of 100 centigrammes, and killed five days after the last dose, no remains of Boric Acid could be found.

On the other hand, it has been pointed out that the method for the chemical quantitative analysis of Boric Acid is far from perfect. This must be conceded. But the quantities used in the preservation of food are so small, that these analytical discrepancies are practically of no account. It has further been objected, that the daily use of different kinds of borated food might disagree with the system; but this objection would only be valid if Borax and Boric Acid were drastic substances with a toxic effect on the organism. Should these substances therefore be discarded solely on the ground of these two unfounded objections, a great check would be given to the progress of national prosperity.

Now, though severest criticism of medical observations, and experience won from experimental research justify the conclusion that Borax and Boric Acid are innocuous as preservatives of food, this assertion of course can only be valid within certain limits, a restriction which however applies to all victuals and drugs; for we know that medicines, admixtures to food, and even aliments, when taken injudiciously or in excess, cease to be wholesome, and suddenly become injurious substances. And moreover, if harm could be done by Borax and Boric Acid used in the preservation of food, the immense quantities which have already been swallowed would have aroused the attention of medical men, particularly as boracic preservation is openly practised (as may be seen by the butchers' trade journals), and has been unreluctantly accepted by the working classes.

For the preservation of meat Boric Acid is used in quantities of $\frac{1}{2}$ to $\frac{3}{4}$ per cent.; of this a great part is lost in watering the meat, particularly in the smoking process for instance, so that we may estimate $\frac{1}{4}$ per cent. as the maximum amount which reaches the system. Experience has proved that 12 decigrammes (1·2 grammes) of Boric Acid or Borax, if taken in food daily, even for a considerable time, does not affect health injuriously. Even quantities twice as large have not been proved injurious, scientific investigations having decisively demonstrated that these doses are far below the limit where deleterious action commences.

Whoever studies the numerous experiments of different investigators with care will end in taking the view of certain authors, a view which has been mentioned above in this discussion, viz., that Borax and Boric Acid, far from being injurious to the human system, are really wholesome substances. But a far greater number of observations will be required before this can be conclusively proved.

Dr. OSCAR LIEBREICH,

o. ö. Professor und Geheimer Medicinalrath.

Berlin,

July, 1899.

APPENDIX No. 1.

Feeding Experiments with Boric Acid on Dogs.

	(a) Yellow Mastiff Bitch.		(b) Poodle (male).	
Date.	Weight. Kilogrammes.	3 grms. Boric Acid per day in 500 cubic centimetres water.	Weight in Kilogrammes.	2 grms. Boric Acid per day in 500 cubic centimetres water.
23 Mar., 1899	12·760		8·530	
27	13·200		8·530	
30	12·400		8·550	
4 April	12·400 (vomiting)		8·530	
6	12·130		8.430 (vomiting)	
10	12·500		8·350	
13	12·570		8·050	
17	12·550		8·270	
21	12·950		7·920	
25	13·020		8·450	
28	13·020		8·520	
Total 36 days.	Weight gained, 20·6 kilogr.	108 grs. Boric Acid fed.	Weight lost, 0·01 kilogr.	72 grms. Boric Acid fed.

(c) Yellow Terrier (male).

Date.	Weight in Kilogrammes.	1 grm. Boric Acid per day in 500 cubic centimetres water.
20 April, 1899	8·520	
25	8·670	
28	8·650	
3 May	9·150	
6	8·870	
9	8·850	
13	8 890	
Total, 24 days.	Gain, 0·370 kilogr.	24 grms. Boric Acid eaten.

APPENDIX No. 2.

(1) Feeding Experiment with Bi-Carbonate of Soda on a Dog.

(*d*) German Mastiff (male).

Date.	Weight in Kilogrammes.	3 grms. in 500 cubic centimetres water daily.
23 Mar., 1899	17·200	
27	18·100	
30	17·800	
4 April	17·300	
6	17·500 (thin stools)	
10	17·400 (thin stools)	
13	17·160	
17	17·100	
21	17·100	
25	17·400	
28	17·150	
Total, 36 days.	Loss, 0·05.	108 grms. bicarbonate of soda fed.

(2) Feeding Experiment with Saltpetre on a Dog.

Hound (male).

Date.	Weight in Kilogrammes.	3 grms. in 500 cubic centimetres water daily.
23 Mar., 1899	27·800	
27	27·400	
30	26·500	
4 April	25·000	
6	23·900 (thin stools)	
10	23·750	
13	23·050	
17	23·000	
21	22·300	
25	22 500	
28	22·400	
Total, 36 days.	Loss, 5·40 = 19·4 per cent.	108 grms. saltpetre fed.

APPENDIX No. 3.

(1) Feeding Experiments with Boric Acid upon Rabbits.

Date.	Grey Rabbit. Weight in grms.	Blue Rabbit. Weight in grms.	Grey Rabbit. Weight in grms.	0·3 grm. Boric Acid in 60 cubic centimetres water per day.
28 Mar., 1899	1370	1270	1170	
4 April	1370	1350	1330	
6	1300	1270	1220	
10	1410	1350	1220	
13	1310	1300	1200	
17	1320	1200	1150	
21	1300	1270	1050	
25	1370	1400	1250	
28	1400	1370	1250	
Total, 31 days.	+ 30 2·2 per cent.	+ 100 7·8 per cent.	+ 80 6·8 per cent.	9·3 grms. Boric Acid fed.

(2) Feeding Experiments with Boric Acid upon Rabbits.

Date.	I.—Grey Rabbit. Weight in grms.	II.—White Rabbit. Weight in grms.	III.—Black Rabbit. Weight in grms.	0·1 grm. Boric Acid in 60 cubic centimetres water per day.
20 April, 1899	1200	1300	1470	
25	1220	1300	1500	
28	1350	1370	1600	
3 May	1240	1370	1580	
6	1270	1350	1700	
9	1250	1330	1650	
13	1270	1370	1630	
Total, 24 days.	+ 70 5·08 per cent.	+ 70 5·4 per cent.	+ 160 10·88 per cent.	2·4 grms. Boric Acid.

(3) Feeding Experiments with Borax upon a Dog.

Black poodle bitch received daily 50 grs. Borax dry in meat.

1 Dec., 1897.	12·200 kilogrs.	
16	13·200 kilogrs.	Blood in stools. Appetite feeble.
17		Violent bleeding.
20		Howls a great deal. Bleeding. Remains in cage. Appetite not diminished.
23		Entirely active.
1 Mar., 1898.	15·620 kilogrs.	

Gain, 3·42 kilogrs. Has taken 450 grs. within 90 days.

(4) Feeding Experiments with Borax upon a Rabbit (weight, 2·400 kilogrammes).

1 Dec., 1898.	5 grms. Borax in 20 cubic centimetres water, poured in by the œsophageal probang.
5	The same dose.

The animal remains absolutely normal.

APPENDIX No. 4.

Feeding Experiments with Borax upon Guinea Pigs.

Three Guinea Pigs received daily 0·5 grm. Borax in 60 cubic centimetres water.

Date.	I.—Weight in grms.	II.—Weight in grms.	III.—Weight in grms.	0·5 grm. Borax in 60 cubic centimetres water per day.
29 Nov., 1897	425	340	330	
2 Dec.	500	440	430	
6	480	420	400	
9	460	375	380	
13	480	420	405	
16	440	365	370	
20	445	400	370	
23	440	350	360	
27	460	380	390	
30	444	365	370	
3 Jan., 1898	446	370	375	
5	420	340	370	
10	395	360	340	
13	405	344	355	
17	400	350	350	
20	390	365	340	
24	395	347	362	
27	415	370	380	
31	422	372	376	
3 Feb.	425	375	370	
7	430	370	373	
11	428	371	375	
15	431	370	376	
19	429	374	378	
22	425	372	374	
25	428	370	379	
28	432	373	381	
3 Mar.	436	377	383	
Total, 95 days.	+ 11	+ 37	+ 53	47·5 grms. Borax fed.

APPENDIX No. 5.

Metabolism Experiment.—Dog. I.

Date.	Weight.	Nitrogenous contents of food.	Urine.				Fæces.			Balance.
			Volume.	Spec. gravity.	Reaction.	Nitrogenous contents.	Fresh	Dry.	Nitrogenous contents.	
A.—Preliminary period.										
7 Mar., 1899	7700	8·749	320	1028	acid	7·078	179	—	—	
8	7710	8·749	306	1030	-	7·111	209	—	—	
9	7680	8·749	210	1028	-	7·056	165	—	—	
10	7650	8·749	250	1030	-	5·700	240	213·5	9·349	
11	7760	8·749	390	1028	-	6·115	189	—	—	
12	7730	8·749	295	1028	-	7·115	208	-	—	
13	7750	8·749	245	1030	-	7·066	146	152·5	6·292	
14	7720	8·749	250	1030	alkal.	5·250	188	—	—	
15	7680	6·749	235	1030	acid	6·843	160	—	—	
16	7630	8·749	220	1031	-	5·289	260	173·0	7·365	
		87·490	2721			64·623	1944	549·0	23·006	—0·139
						23·006				
						87·629				
B.—Borax period. 20 grs. Borax daily.										
17 Mar., 1899	7650	8·749	172	1044	alkal.	6·020	138	—	—	
18	7620	8·749	158	1044	-	4·734	121	—	—	
19	7690	8·749	198	1042	-	5·655	190	—	—	
20	7750	8·749	275	1039	-	6·083	141	590	11·301	
21	7800	8·749	240	1039	-	5·040	182	-	—	
22	7800	8·749	215	1039	-	5·599	139	—	—	
23	7790	8·749	195	1039	-	5·078	152	473	9·020	
24	7770	8·749	280	1036	-	6·350	191	—	—	
25	7720	8·749	370	1034	-	6·112	175	—	—	
26	7700	8·749	290	1038	-	5·846	205	571	11·014	
		87·490	2393			56·517	1634	504	31·335	—0·362
						31·335				
						87·852				
C.—After period.										
29 April, 1899	7710	8·749	260	1038	alkal.	6·625	162	—	—	
30	7750	8·749	230	1039	-	6·054	182	—	—	
1 May	7820	8·749	220	1040	-	6·703	193	—	—	
2	7880	8·749	195	1040	-	6·716	190	200·5	9·764	
3	7850	8·749	165	1041	-	4·943	205	—	—	
4	7870	8·749	290	1034	-	6·538	228	—	—	
5	7850	8·749	85	1041	-	7·589	176	171·0	8·312	
6	7830	8·749	255	1036	-	8·568	190	—	—	
7	7790	8·749	100	1040	-	3·284	137	—	—	
8	7750	8·749	152	1040	-	5·107	225	156·5	7·651	
		87·490	1952			62·127	1888	528·0	25·727	—0·464
						25·727				
						87·954				

APPENDIX No. 6.

Influence of Borax, Carbonate of Soda, and Saltpetre on Salival Ferment.

Into each of a number of small flasks, 10 cubic centimetres of mixed human saliva, obtained by subcutaneous injection, were introduced, then solutions of Borax, carbonate of soda, and saltpetre, as well as 20 cubic centimetres $2\frac{1}{2}$ per cent. decoction of starch added, together with water enough to make 100 cubic centimetres. After standing at 122° Fahr. for an hour, then boiled, the sugar which had formed in each flask was determined.

A.

Small Flask	I.	II.	III.	IV.	V.	VI.	VII.
	Borax.		Carbonate of Soda		Saltpetre.		Control.
Admixture of ..	0·1	0·5	0·1	0·5	0·1	0·5	
Sugar	0·164	0·158	traces	0·0	0·207	0·229	0·2075

The same arrangement, but the flasks, after having stood for an hour at 122° Fahr., were only boiled up after 20 hours.

B.

Small Flasks.	VIII.	IX.	X.	XI.	XII.	XIII.	XIV.
	Borax.		Carbonate of Soda		Saltpetre.		Control.
Admixture of ..	0·1	0·5	0·1	0·5	0·1	0·5	
Sugar	0·204	0·205	0·210	0·0805	0·208	0·256	0·249

APPENDIX No. 7.

Artificial Digestion-Experiments with Borax, Boric Acid, and Saltpetre.

0·5 grm. Pepsine, 0·8 grm. hydrochloric acid, and 0·5 grm. albumen were put into each of several small flasks; then solutions of *Borax* (neutralised by $\frac{1}{10}$ *normal hydrochloric acid*), Boric Acid and saltpetre were added, and water added to make 100 cubic centimetres. The flasks were left standing for 24 hours at 98·6° Fahr.

I.—Borax.

Small Flask.	I.	II.	III.	IV.
Admixture of Borax ..	0·1	0·25	0·5	Control-experiment.
Neutralised with $\frac{1}{10}$ normal hydrochloric acid	5·3	13·25	26·5	0·0
Digested	Entirely	Entirely	Small residuum	Entirely.

II.—Boric Acid.

I.	II.	III.	IV.	V.	VI.	VII.	VIII.	IX.	X.
0·1	0·25	0·5	1·0	1·5	2·0	2·5	4·0	4·5	5·0

After 24 hours at 98·6° Fahr., *perfect digestion* in *each case.*

III.—Saltpetre.

Small Flasks.	I.	II.	III.	IV.
Admixture of Saltpetre	0·1	0·2	0·5	1·0
Digested after 24 hours	$\frac{3}{4}$	$\frac{1}{2}$	—	—

APPENDIX No. 8.

Action of Borax, Boric Acid, Carbonate of Soda, and Saltpetre on Extract of Pancreas.

The pancreatic gland of a pig, weighing 110 grms., after being rubbed down with sand and powdered glass, was left to digest for an hour in 550 cubic centimetres water; 50 cubic centimetres of the filtrate was mixed with different salt solutions, 30 cubic centimetres of a decoction of starch was added, and the whole brought to 150 cubic centimetres by addition of water. Left to stand for 24 hours at 98·6° Fahr.; then, after separation of the albuminoid bodies, the quantity of sugar formed was determined.

Small Flasks.	I.	II.	III.	IV.	V.
	Borax.			Boric Acid.	
Admixture of	1·0	2·0	3·0	2·5	5·0
Glucose found.. ..	0·768	0·770	0·753	0·790	0·789

Small Flasks.	VI.	VII.	VIII.	IX.	X.
	Carbonate of Soda.		Nitrate of Potash.		Control-experiment.
Admixture of ..	0·5	1·0	0·5	1·0	—
Glucose found ..	0·530	0·355	0·790	0·785	0·791

APPENDIX No. 9.

Action of Borax, Boric Acid, Carbonate of Soda, and Saltpetre on Emulsine.

0·5 emulsine was put into a number of small flasks and brayed with solutions of weighed quantities of Boric Acid, Borax, saltpetre, and anhydric carbonate of soda; then the weighed amygdaline added, and water added to make 100 cubic centimetres. Left to stand for 48 hours at 100·4° Fahr., and then acidified by sulphuric acid; then distilled into receivers previously charged with liquor potassæ, and the prussic acid titrated in the distillate by means of a solution of silver.

Small Flasks.	I.	II.	III.	IV.	V.	VI.
	Boric Acid.					
Admixture of	0·5	1·0	2·0	2·5	4·0	5·0
Amygdaline	1·583	1·513	1·561	1·612	1·690	1·659
Prussic acid found	0·0919	0·0874	0·0898	0·0929	0.0972	0·0956
Prussic acid calculated . .	0·0937	0·0894	0·0922	0·0952	0·0999	0·0980
In per cent.	98·0	97·8	97·4	97·5	97·3	97·5

Small Flasks.	VII.	VIII.	IX.	X.	XI.	XII.	XIII.	XIV.
	Borax.			Saltpetre.		Carbonate of Soda.		Control experiment.
Admixture of . .	1·0	2·0	3·0	0·25	0·5	0·5	1·0	—
Amygdaline . .	1·672	1·578	1·582	1·557	1·427	1·855	1·844	1·461
Prussic acid found	0·0162	0·0105	0·0082	0·0773	0·0729	0·0054	0·0027	0·0848
Prussic acid calculated.	0·0988	0·0932	0·0935	0·0920	0·0843	0·1096	0·1089	0·0863
In per cent. . .	16·4	11·3	8·8	86·8	83·8	4·9	2·5	98·2

APPENDIX No. 10.

Experiments on the influence of Boric Acid, Borax (anhydric), Soda (anhydric), Saltpetre, and Common Salt on the gastric and intestinal epithelia of Dogs.

Dogs were narcotised by means of morphine hydrochloride and ether, the stomach laid open and evacuated, and parts of it irrigated for five minutes with the solutions mentioned. The small intestine was divided into separate parts by ligatures, without injuring the afferent bloodvessels. The divisions were filled with the different liquids without much tension. Opened after five minutes. Mucous membrane excised and examined in a fresh state under the microscope. For further microscopical examination fresh pieces of the gastric and intestinal mucous membranes were fixed and hardened in absolute alcohol, then embedded in paraffin. The sections coloured with hæmatoxyline (nuclear staining) and eosine, and mounted in Canada balsam.

EXAMINATION OF THE STOMACH.

Percentage.	Boric Acid.	Borax.	Soda.	Saltpetre.	Common Salt.
½	—	Gastric mucous membrane remains **perfectly normal**	Mucous membrane becomes paler immediately, otherwise **normal**	Remains **normal**	—
1	Mucous membrane, **normal**	Very slight pallor, otherwise **normal**	Mucous membrane immediately becomes quite pale	Distinct pallor immediately, increasing during irrigation	—
2	Mucus of a whitish colour	Some increase of pallor	Mucous membrane immediately becomes very pale	Greater pallor than with the 1 per cent. solution	—
3	Mucous membrane seems lightly veiled	Still paler; somewhat swollen	Ditto	Ditto, white spots where the solution impinges on the membrane	Mucous membrane a uniform pink colour
5	Mucous membrane shows no effect, **normal**	Ditto	Mucous membrane paler than with the other concentrations	All symptoms become more distinct	Ditto

APPENDIX No. 11.

Microscopic Appearances of the Fresh Gastric Mucous Membrane.

Percentage.	Boric Acid.	Borax.	Soda.	Saltpetre.	Common Salt.
½		The free surface remains perfectly **normal**	No change recognisable **normal**	Cells **normal**	
1	Gastric mucous membrane **normal**	ditto **normal**	The free surface of the mucous membrane is somewhat translucent and covered by a layer of cast epithelial cells, which are modified in the same way as by an admixture of caustic soda solution. The epithelium, which still remains fixed on the surface, shows no discernible alteration	Here and there are found a few swollen cells projecting dome-like beyond the free surface of the epithelium Only these cells are turbid	
2	**Normal**	The greater part of the epithelial cells are **normal**. Some are swollen up and translucent. They are more easily detachable from the foundation, and are mingled with the slightly increased layer of mucus	The same changes, but more cast off cells. The transparency and shedding of the cells goes on to a greater depth in the mucous membrane than before	In most places no alteration of the epithelial layer is observable. Only the topmost layers show a number of swollen cells ; the latter are dome-shaped, turbid, and highly granulated	

APPENDIX No. 11—*continued.*

Percentage.	Boric Acid.	Borax.	Soda.	Saltpetre.	Common Salt.
3	**Normal**	Changes of the same kind and degree	Kind and degree of change the same as in 2 per cent. solution	With low-power magnification the epithelial layers of the mucous membrane appear less transparent than they are normally. With high magnifying power an intense granular turbidity of the epithelial cells is seen. The latter have lost their characteristic cylindrical shape; some of them look like misshapen bales. But they are still connected one with the other, and have only lost their cell boundaries at many places	**Normal**
5	**Normal**	Ditto, only the inter-cellular connection in some places is greatly swollen	The surface is destroyed to such a depth that on the normal glands below there lies a layer of matted hæmoglobinous masses in which cells can be hardly recognised	The same changes	**Normal**

APPENDIX No. 12.

Stomach, Microscopically Examined in Hardened Preparations.

Percentage.	Boric Acid.	Borax.	Soda.	Saltpetre.	Common Salt.
½		Perfectly **normal**	Exposed cell-membrane completely obliterated, **otherwise normal**	Free surface of cells coagulated. Border irregular	
1	Mucous membrane perfectly **normal**	Free border of cells considerably shorter, boundaries indistinct, plentiful deposit of mucus	Cell - boundaries obliterated. Numerous cells have been cast off and are superposed on the mucous membrane, forming a separate layer	The border is less even and the cells project dome-like; otherwise the cells are distinctly preserved	
2	A slight layer of mucus discernible on the cells, which in other respects are **normal**	Essentially the same. In the mucus-layer there are a few solitary cells that have been shed	Cells irregular, have become quite low. Cell-boundaries obliterated. On the surface a layer partly albuminous and partly mucous	Cells have become lower. On the surface there is granulated substance, probably albumen (since it is stained red)	
3	Surface entirely normal All cells well preserved. A trace of mucus-layer	The same as in a 2 per cent. solution	The same appearance as before. On the surface a thick albuminous layer. The sub-mucous vessels greatly congested	The cells become irregular in height; otherwise same as above	Slight accumulations of mucus on the surface of the cells, **otherwise normal**
5	Surface **perfectly normal**	The upper portion of the epithelial cells is detached and lies separate on the top of the remaining mucous membrane	Surface cells in some places completely shed; otherwise same as in the 3 per cent. solution	The same as before. There is also a layer of mucus	Slight irregularities on the surface

APPENDIX No. 13.

Microscopic Inspection of the Intestine.

Percentage.	Boric Acid.	Borax.	Soda.	Saltpetre.	Common Salt.
$\frac{1}{2}$		Mucous membrane remains normal	Mucous membrane paler, otherwise normal	Mucous membrane normal, slightly paler	
1	Mucous membrane hardly paler	Ditto	Mucous membrane pale and slightly swollen	Ditto	
2	Mucous membrane very little paler	Ditto slightly reddened	Mucous membrane more swollen, pale pink, and succulent	Mucous membrane a little paler, normal	
3	Mucous membrane somewhat paler	Ditto normal	More swollen than with 2 per cent. solution. Redder and more succulent	Very little paler than normal	Mucous membrane smooth The individual cells indistinct, but still recognisable
5	Mucous membrane much paler, normal	Ditto redder	Mucous membrane much reddened, much swollen and extremely succulent	Very red and succulent	Mucous membrane pale, smooth, and swollen, the individual cells not recognisable

APPENDIX No. 14.

Microscopic Appearance of the Intestinal Mucous Membrane.

Percentage.	Boric Acid.	Borax.	Soda.	Saltpetre.	Common Salt.
½		Epithelium perfectly normal	Epithelium normal	Epithelium normal	
1	Mucous membrane normal	In some places slight swelling of the mucous membrane, so that the margin of its surface looks slightly irregular	A small number of the epithelial cells have been shed, and these are slightly swollen	Ditto	
2	Ditto	Ditto	Many cells disintegrated and swollen. In many places the epithelial cells are still attached and, where so, they are normal	The epithelial cells are normal	
3	Ditto	Ditto	Same as with 2 per cent. solution, but more intense	Epithelial cells a little swollen, margin irregular, cells slightly granulated and turbid, cell-boundaries somewhat indistinct	Epithelium normal
5	Normal	Ditto	Almost all structure has disappeared. The cells are disintegrated macerated, swollen, and translucent. Shape of any kind can hardly be discerned. The action extends in some parts as low down as the cell-stroma	The epithelial cells are swollen, the outer margin irregular, the cells much granulated and turbid, and the boundaries indistinct	Normal

APPENDIX No. 15.

Hardened Preparation of the Intestine examined under the Microscope.

Per-centage.	Boric Acid.	Borax.	Soda.	Saltpetre.	Common Salt.
½		Cells **normal** A slightly thicker coating of mucus on the surface	**Normal**	A very small number of disintegrated cells.	
1	Mucous membrane **normal**	The cells at the surface form a matted layer. Nuclei **normal**. The border margin has disappeared	Cells disintegrated in numbers. Cell - boundary has dis appeared. Nuclei **normal**	Ditto.	
2	Ditto	Same as with 1 per cent. solution	Cells cast off in numbers. Cells at the surface mixed with mucus and albumen	Cells cast off in numbers. The epithelial cells swollen on the surface and somewhat irregular	
3	Ditto	Same as with 1 per cent. solution	The cells are covered with a thick layer of albuminous mucus and disintegrated cells	Ditto, somewhat stronger	Mucous membrane perfectly **normal**
5	**Normal**	Cells disintegrated in great numbers. Nuclei everywhere distinctly visible	Ditto	Nearly the entire protoplasmic layer is destroyed.	**Normal**; in some places the secretion of mucus slightly increased.

LITERATURE.

1. BINSWANGER, L. "Pharmakologische Würdigung der Borsäure, des Borax und anderer borsauren Verbindungen in ihrer Einwirkung auf den gesunden und kranken thierischen Organismus." München, 1847.

2. LISTER, J. "On Recent Improvements in the Details of Antiseptic Surgery." *The Lancet*, 1st May, 1875, p. 603 *et seq.*

3. CANE, L. "On Boracic Acid and Ordinary Dressing for Wounds." *The Lancet*, 1876, p. 734.

4. BEZOLD, FR. "Ueber die Borsäurebehandlung bei Mittelohreiterungen und die gegen dieselbe erhobenen Einwürfe." *Deutsche med. Wochenschrift*, No. 8, 1887, p. 147.

5. GOWERS, W. R. "On Psoriasis from Borax." *The Lancet*, 1881, Vol. II., p. 546.

6. EVANS, J. JAMESON. "Toxic Effects of Boracic Acid." *British Medical Journal*, No. 1987, 28th January, 1899, p. 209.

7. GRUMPELT, SOPHIA. "Symptoms of Poisoning by Boracic Acid." *British Medical Journal*, No. 1984, 7th January, 1899, p. 17.

8. MOLODENKOW. "2 Fälle von Vergiftung durch Borsäure" (Wratsch No. 31). *Petersburger med. Wochenschrift*, No. 42, 1881.

9. LEMOINE, G. "De la toxicité de l'Acide borique." *Gazette médicale de Paris*, No. 18, 1890, p. 205.

10. BRUZELIUS, R. "Om Borsyreförgiftning." Hygiea, 1882, p. 548. Ref. in *Virchow-Hirsch Jahresbericht*, 1883, Vol. I., p. 400.

11. WARFWINGE, F. W. "Fall af Borsyreförgiftning." *Sv. läkaresällsk. förhandl.*, 1883, p. 10. Ref. in *Virchow-Hirsch Jahresbericht*, 1883, Vol. I., p. 401.

12. HOGNER, R. "Förgiftningsfall genom Borsyresköljningar." Eira, 1884, p. 389. Ref. in *Virchow-Hirsch Jahresbericht*, 1884, Vol. I., p. 359.

13. RASCH, C. "Ein Fall von Borsäure-Exanthem." Hospitalstidende, 1897, p. 709. Ref. in *Virchow-Hirsch Jahresbericht*, 1897, p. 351.

14. WELCH, G. T "Toxicological Effects of Boracic Acid." *New York Medical Record*, 3rd November, 1888 p. 531. Ref. in *Virchow-Hirsch Jahresbericht*, 1888, Vol. I., p. 354.

15 BRÜCKE, M. E. "Ueber das Verhalten einiger Eiweisskörper gegen Borsäure." Sitzungsber. d. K. Akademie d. Wiss. zu Wien, 1867. No. 55, Vol. II., p. 881.

16. LIEBREICH, O. "Ueber Conservirung durch Borsäure." *Berl. klin. Wochenschr.*, No. 33, 1887, p. 605.

"The putting into execution of methods intended for the preservation or substitution of food stuffs, is nowadays rendered far more difficult than was formerly the case. Who would have made the introduction of pickled meat, smoked meat, and such like, dependent upon a chemical or pharmacological investigation?"

17. BAUMERT, G. "Zur Frage des normalen Vorkommens der Borsäure im Weine." Ber. d. deutsch. chem. Gesellsch., 1888, No. XXI., p. 3290.

18. JAY, H. "La Dispersion de l'Acide borique." Ann. d'Hygiène, 1896, tome 35, No. 1, p. 23. Compt. rend., 1895, 121, p. 896.

19. LEGENDRE. "Traité pratique d'Antisepsie appliqué à la Thérapeutique et à l'Hygiène." Paris, 1888, p. 72.

20. POLLI, H. "Applicazioni terapeutiche dell' Acido borico." *Gaz. med. Italiana, Lombardia*, No. 26, 1877, p. 254. Citat aus Ber. d. deutsch. chem. Gesellsch, 1877. X², p. 1382.

21. VIRCHOW, R. "Ueber Nephritis arthritica." *Berl. klin. Wochenschr.* No. 1, 1884.

"Als ich diese Massen von Krystallen vor mir sah (im Urin), war mein erster Gedanke: da muss doch ein energisches alkalisches Regime helfen. Ich fuhr nach Hause und gleich am Nachmittag füllte ich mich mit einer starken Dose von borsaurem Natron, nahm am nächsten Morgen Karlsbader Wasser, und von da ab habe ich nie wieder Erscheinungen ähnlicher Art gehabt Ich fuhr 3 Monate lang mit meinem alkalischen Regime fort, und bis auf den heutigen Tag habe ich niemals wieder Eiter abgesondert, noch Albumen, noch Cylinder producirt; mein Harn ist so klar wie der einer Jungfrau. Ich kann sagen, dass ich selbst überrascht gewesen bin durch diese acute Wandlung."

22. NEUMANN, J. "Experimentelle Untersuchungen über die Wirkung der Borsäure." Inaug.-Dissert. Dorpat, 1879, und Arch. f. exp. Path. u. Pharm., No. 14, 1881, p. 149.

23. GRUBER, M. "Ueber den Einfluss des Borax auf die Eiweisszersetzung im Organismus. *Zeitschrift für Biologie*, No. 16, 1880, p. 198.

24. DE CYON, E. "Sur l'Action Physiologique du Borax." Compt. rend., 1878, tome 87, p. 845.

25. FORSTER, J. "Ueber die Verwendbarkeit der Borsäure zur Conservirung von Nahrungsmitteln." *Archiv für Hygiene*, 1884, Vol. II., p. 75.

26. CHITTENDEN, R. H., and GIES, WILLIAM J. "The Influence of Borax and Boric Acid upon Nutrition, with special reference to Proteid Metabolism." *The American Journal of Physiology*, 3rd January, 1898, Vol. I, p. 1.

27. CHITTENDEN, R. H. "Influence du Borax et de l'Acide borique sur la Digestion." *Gazette de Diététique et d'Hygiène*, New York, February, 1893, citirt aus: Avis des Savants et Médecins, Flers-de-L'orne, 1896.

28. KEPPLER, F. "Ueber den Wirkungswerth von Pepsin und Pankreatin bei Gegenwart von Borsäure." *Pharmaceutische Centralhalle*, 1899, No. 2, p. 17.

29. BROUARDEL. "Intoxication par Produits journellement absorbés à petite dose." 4. Congrès international d'Hygiène et de Démographie. Genève, 1882, Vol. II., p. 352.

The Society for the protection of the interests of the German chemical industry, recently in session at Frankfort, has unanimously passed a resolution against the prohibition of the use of boric acid for the preservation of meats, and has appealed to the Bundesrath to reverse its decision. Science N.S. XV. No. 405. p. 559.

EXPLANATION OF THE ILLUSTRATIONS.

PLATE 1.

Fig. 1. Section of a *normal* stomach. The Epithelium is completely preserved, the nuclei lie at the basis of the cells. The separate cells are distinctly defined. The free surface presents a smooth appearance, no cells projecting above it.

Fig. 2. ½ per cent. *Borax*, no change as compared with Fig. 1. (Stomach.)

Fig. 3. 1 per cent. *Borax*. The cells are shorter than normal. The cell boundaries indistinct and vague. (Stomach.)

Fig. 4. 5 per cent. *Boric Acid*. Stomach also normal. No effect can be perceived.

Fig. 5. ½ per cent. *Soda*. The cell boundaries faded. (Stomach.)

Fig. 6. 1 per cent. *Soda*. The cell boundaries are faded, disintegrated cell-substance on the surface. (Stomach.)

PLATE 2.

Fig. 7. 5 per cent. Saltpetre. Shows an extremely powerful effect. The cell boundaries are preserved wherever the cells are preserved; in some places, however, the epithelium is completely destroyed; on the surface there is a mass of mucus mixed with blood. (Stomach.)

Fig. 8. *Normal Intestine*. The surface shows a cuticular layer with double contour, some goblet-cells are to be seen, the nuclei lie at the basis of the cells. The cell boundaries are visible, but they are not so distinct as in the stomach.

Fig. 9. 5 per cent. *Boric Acid*. No change from the normal appearance. (Intestine.)

Fig. 10. 2 per cent. *Borax*. The cell boundaries are perhaps a little less distinct in some places. The marginal border no longer visible?

Fig. 11. 2 per cent. *Soda*. In the space between two intestinal villi lie numerous disintegrated cells, which come from another portion of the epithelium.

Fig. 12. 5 per cent. *Saltpetre*. The free surface of the cells is destroyed, the cuticular layer has disappeared, the free surface has a fringed appearance. (Intestine.)

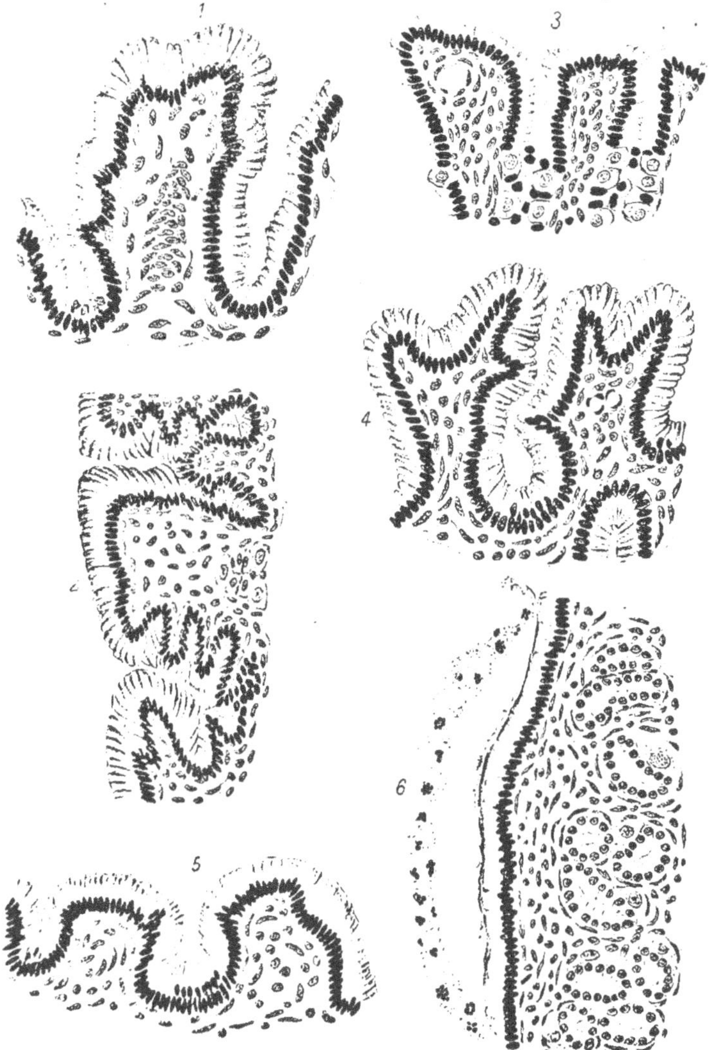

fec. Paul i Gunther

7

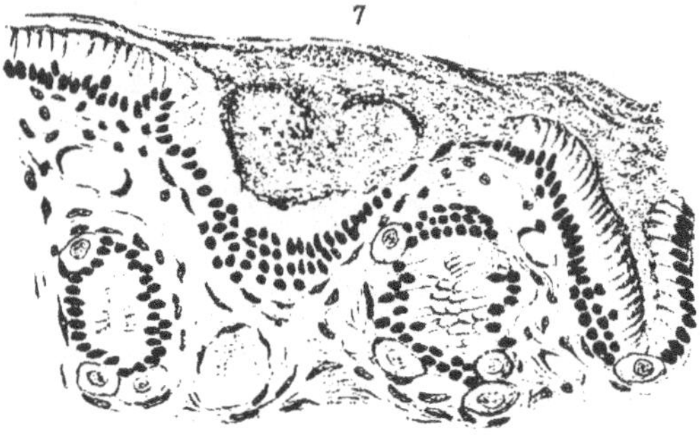

8

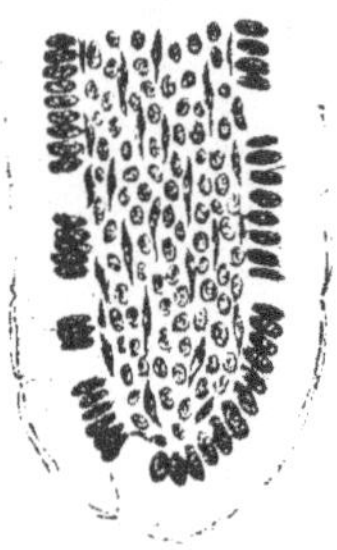

9

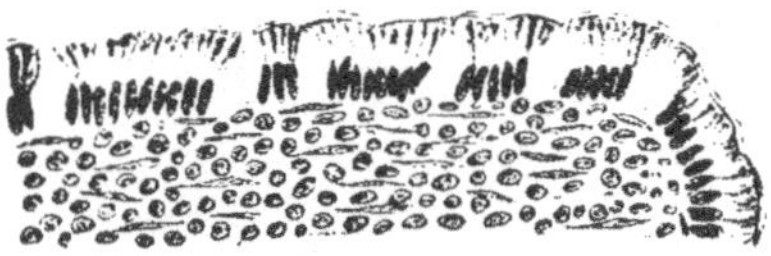

10

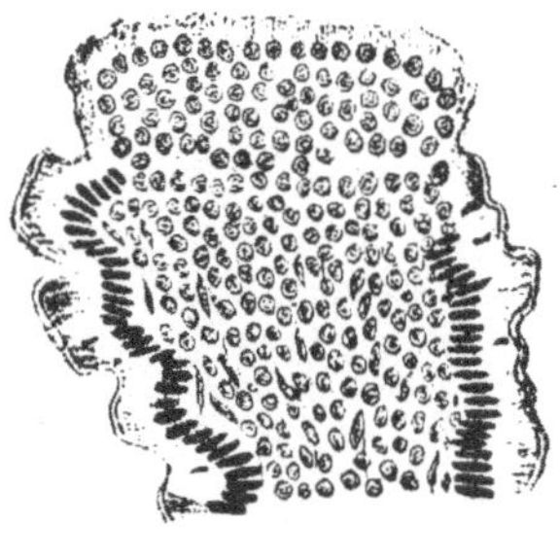

11

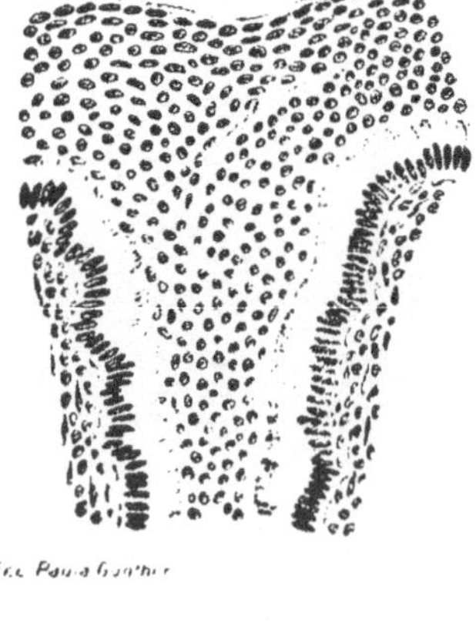

12

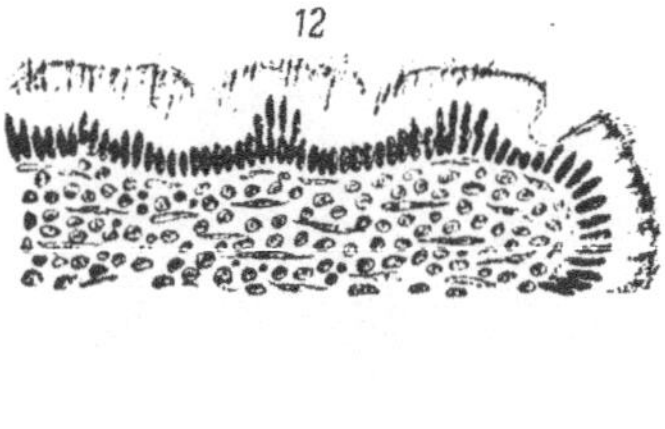

fec. Paula Günther

Spotted something that isn't quite right?

Let us know and we'll fix it for future reprints. And as a thank you for your diligence, we'll send you a free Sothis book of your choice.

publisher@sothis.press

This page intentionally left blank

Except of course for that line above. And this one.
And whilst we have your attention, perhaps you'd
like to follow us on Instagram @sothis.press. Go on.

Made in United States
Cleveland, OH
05 November 2026

47667155R00038